Lifestyle Medicine

Cooper Wellness Center

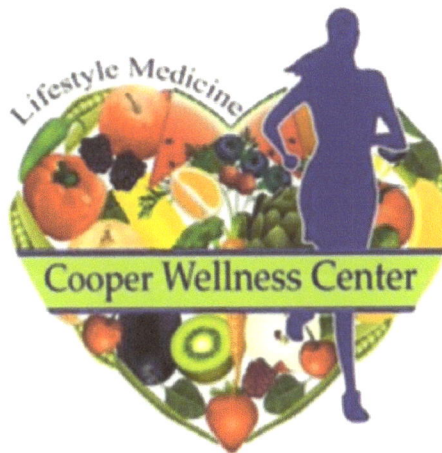

Wellness Program Manual

Cooper Wellness and Disease Prevention Center
3604 N. McColl Rd. McAllen, TX 78501
www.CooperWellnessCenter.com

Printed in the United States of America.
ISBN: 978-0-9973379-3-8 (paperback)
ISBN: 978-0-9973379-5-2 (eBook)

CONTENTS

Welcome to Wellness!

We are excited that you have chosen to join the Cooper Wellness & Disease Prevention Center Wellness Program. The Texas Rio Grande Valley is experiencing a near epidemic of chronic diseases. As many as half of the people in the Valley will develop *diabetes* in their lifetime. The Valley tops the *obesity* list in the nation. In addition, one in every three women and one in every two men in the Valley will develop *cancer* in their lifetime. We are committed to REDUCING and IMPROVING our patients' conditions through lifestyle medicine.

Our medical director, Dr. Dona Cooper-Dockery is board certified in Internal Medicine. Her broad range of experience and training allows her to treat a variety of medical conditions in the Wellness Center. She says, "as a practicing physician for over 22 years, I have become uncomfortable with only prescribing pills." We are glad that you have joined the journey to embrace life-changing methods to **reduce** or **reverse** chronic disease. Our treatments and wellness programs include one-on-one and group lifestyle coaching, exercise sessions and diet modification strategies combined with hydrotherapy and other therapy treatments.

Wellness Is A Choice

Our Wellness program has been designed as a result of years of research into the causes of chronic diseases. Lifestyle medicine is the emerging, cutting edge approach that is achieving phenomenal results. You will discover that not only will your physical health improve, but your mental and spiritual outlook will also improve.

"Good health and wellness is a choice not destiny!"
-Dr. Dona Cooper-Dockery, Medical Director, Cooper Wellness & Disease Prevention Center

This workbook contains material that will be reviewed as you go through the various classes and programs here at the Cooper Wellness and Disease Prevention Center. Feel free to address any questions you may have to one of our staff members. Once again, welcome.

Frequently Asked Questions

Emergencies: The Cooper Wellness Center operates between the hours of 8:30 am to 5:30 pm Monday through Friday. Our staff is available for your care during the above hours. In case of emergency, call our central telephone line 956-627-3106 and the answering service will record your message. If it is an emergency, call 911.

Fitness Center: Each guest will be placed on an individual fitness program that involves equipment in our state-of-the art Fitness Center. When using the Fitness Center, we encourage you to talk with one of our fitness coaches for proper instruction using the aerobic equipment.

Food: We prefer that all food is consumed in the designated dining area. Eating food at times other than what is outlined in your program will interfere with the principles being taught in the program, except when the physician orders additional supplementation.

Leaving the Wellness Center: Leaving the Wellness Center for any reason other than the completion of your session is usually not in the best interest of a health guest as it interrupts the program's continuity. However, if you find you need to leave please notify the staff so we will know when to expect your return.

Program Evaluation: Your evaluation of this program is very important to us. We would appreciate your taking time to complete a Wellness Program questionnaire before you leave. The information that you provide will be of benefit to future programs. Thank you for taking the time!

Research: Your participation in our research study will help us objectively to assess the influence of the wellness program on our guests' health habits. When you consent to the research project, data gathered from our guests' responses on lifestyle practices will be used to evaluate the objectives of our program.

Phone: There are courtesy phones in the Lounge and the Education Classroom. The Wellness Center number is 956-627-3106.

Wellness Program Packages

All Wellness Program Packages Include:

- ❖ Guidance Manual
- ❖ Initial physician medical consultation with labs, body fat analysis and health risk assessment
- ❖ Personalized goal and plan development customized to get results, including monitoring of your progress
- ❖ Weekly visit with your provider
- ❖ Weekly Wellness Program group sessions on-site & access to weekly lectures and special guest presentations
- ❖ Weekly one-on-one telephone coaching with your personal lifestyle coach
- ❖ Nutrition & exercise journal
- ❖ Supplements & vitamins for program's duration (30 days)
- ❖ Incredibly Delicious Vegan Recipes & Meal Plans Cookbook ($32.00 value)
- ❖ Weekly Healthy Cooking classes
- ❖ Two weekly fitness trainer-supervised exercise sessions on cite in our state-of-the-art Fitness Center
- ❖ Weekly hydrotherapy, massage therapy, light therapy and sauna therapy treatment options
- ❖ Future, on-going support available (please inquire about fee)

4-Week to Wellness Program
Designed as an overview to kick-start your lifestyle transformation efforts

8-Week to Wellness Program.
For greater depth of knowledge and deeper commitment

12-Week Get Healthy for Life Program
For TOTAL commitment to reducing and reversing chronic disease

Wellness Program Kick-Off

Step 1: Call the Cooper Wellness Center (CWC) at 956-627-3106 to speak with a lifestyle coach who will briefly review your goals, needs and enroll you as a Wellness program participant.

Step 2: Come to the CWC to complete your pre-program lab work, body fat analysis & Health Risk Assessment.

Step 3: You will have your initial medical consultation with the physician to review your assessment results. Your personal lifestyle coach will also give you an orientation to the program.

Step 4: You are on your way to lifestyle transformation. Join us at your weekly group session, come exercise and enjoy a healthy cooking class! We'll be calling to check in with you about your progress along the way.

Step 5: Graduation! Continuation of your wellness journey and your new life....

ASSESS YOUR HEALTH STATUS
HOW HEALTHY ARE YOU?

HOW HEALTHY IS YOUR LIFESTYLE?

INSTRUCTIONS: For each health indicator, check the box in the column that best describes you. Write the score for that column in the Score column on the right.

HEALTH INDICATORS	COLUMN A 0	COLUMN B 5	COLUMN C 10	SCORE
1. **Disease –** do you have high blood pressure?	Yes, uncontrolled	Yes, controlled	No	_____
2. **Disease –** do you have diabetes?	Yes, uncontrolled	Yes, controlled	No	_____
3. **Disease –** do you have heart disease?	Yes, uncontrolled	Yes, controlled	No	_____
4. **Body weight -** What is your body mass index?	BMI 30+	BMI 25-29.9	BMI <25	_____
5. **Blood Pressure –** What is your blood pressure?	140/90+	120/80-139/89	<120/80	_____
6. **Physical Activity** – Do you engage in at least 30 minutes daily of moderate or vigorous exercise?	No regular physical exercise	2-3 days per week	5-7 days per week	_____

7. **Fruits and vegetables -** How many daily servings do you consume? (1 serving =1 medium fruit, ½ c. cooked vegetables or 1 c. raw vegetables.)	0-3		4-5	6-9	____
HEALTH INDICATORS	**COLUMN A** 0	**COLUMN B** 5	**COLUMN C** 10	**SCORE**	
8. **Whole grains** – How many servings per day do you consume? (1 serving=1 slice whole wheat bread, 2/3 c. brown rice, oatmeal, quinoa or dry cereal)	<1/day	1-2 servings/ day	3+ servings/ day	____	
9. **Legumes** - How many servings of legumes do you have per day? (1/2 c. cooked beans, peas, lentils)	<1 servings per day	1-2 servings per day	3 or more servings per day	____	
10. **Nuts seeds -** How many servings do you have per week. (1 servings =1 oz. nuts or seeds, 2 tbsp. of nut butter)	0-2 servings per week	2- 4 servings per week	5 or more servings per week	____	
11. **Red and Processed meats-** How many servings of meat do you have per day? (egg, beef, ham, sausage, salami; 1 serving = 3oz.)	> 3 servings per day	1-2 servings per day	< 1 serving per day	____	

12. **Snack foods** - How many times per week do you consume candy bars, chips, fries, sodas, etc..	>7 times per week	2-6 times per week	<1 per week	____	
13. **Water** - How many cups of water do you drink daily?	<5 cups per day	6-7 cups per day	8 or more cups per day	____	
HEALTH INDICATORS	**COLUMN A** 0	**COLUMN B** 5	**COLUMN C** 10	**SCORE**	
14. **Breakfast** - Do you have breakfast regularly?	seldom	sometimes	daily	____	
15. **Sleep** - Average hours of sleep per day.	<6 hours per day	< 7hours or more per day	>8 hours per day	____	
16. **Sugar** - What is your blood sugar level, if known?	126+	100-125	<100	____	
17. *Blood Cholesterol* - What is your LDL cholesterol level?	160+	130-159	<130	____	
18. *Smoking Status* -Indicate your present status.	current smoker	ex-smoker	non-smoker	____	
HEALTH INDICATORS	**COLUMN A** 0	**COLUMN B** 5	**COLUMN C** 10	**SCORE**	

19. **Social relationships -** Indicate your status.	Have no social or family support/ rarely connect	Some family and social support/ connect occasionally	Strong family and social support/ frequently connect	____
20. **Happiness** - How happy are you?	Not happy, often sad or depressed	Somewhat happy/ seldom sad	Very happy and satisfied with life	____
21. **Time outdoors** - How much time do you spend outdoors?	< 10 min. per day	10-30 min. per day	30 min. or more per day	____
22. **Hope and the future -** What is your outlook about the future?	Pessimistic	Somewhat optimistic	Very optimistic	____
23. **Spiritual connection/ meditation -** Indicate your status.	No spiritual or religious belief; I do not meditate	I am learning about spiritual values/ I meditate often	I have faith and engage regularly with people of the same faith/ I meditate regularly	____

Total Lifestyle Score: _____

0-60 very high risk	65-100 moderate risk	105-150 average risk	155-200 good	205-300 excellent

PERSONAL GOALS

Check or select all the changes you wish to implement that will promote better personal health.

- ☐ Achieve and maintain a healthier weight
- ☐ Improve or reverse diabetes
- ☐ Improve or reverse hypertension
- ☐ Improve overall health
- ☐ Reduce medications
- ☐ Improve physical endurance
- ☐ Eat at least eight servings of fruits and vegetables daily
- ☐ Eat at least five servings of whole grains weekly
- ☐ Reduce the consumption of processed or refined foods
- ☐ Increase the intake of nuts and seeds
- ☐ Get at least thirty minutes of physical exercise daily, a minimum of six days weekly
- ☐ Get seven to eight hours of timely rest per night
- ☐ Spend more time with family and friends
- ☐ Have devotional exercise or meditation at least twenty to thirty minutes per day
- ☐ To live disease free for life

MY COMMITMENT

It is my deepest desire to implement the changes listed above as I embrace all of the knowledge I will gain during this Wellness program.

Signed by:_____Date:_____

Week 1: State of health in the world

Week 2: Evaluating your lifestyle

Week 3: Program of Behavioral change

Week 4: Impact of health environment

HEALTH EDUCATION

What is Health Education? Many answers have been given to this question; however, three definitions have been chosen that must be remembered.

> First, the World Health Organization (WHO) state that it "comprises consciously constructed opportunities for learning involving some form of communication designed to improve health literacy, including improving knowledge, and developing life skills which are conducive to individual and community health".

> Likewise, Lawrence W. Green conceptualizes it as "an interactive process that facilitates voluntary changes in health behaviors, through the combination of planned learning experiences".

> According to Alessandro Sepilli, "it is the educational process that tends to hold citizens individually and collectively in the defense of their own health and that of others."

Consequently, Health Education is a process of lifelong learning, aimed at promoting living conditions that help people to have a good state of health and thus reduce the risks of illness and death.

Why is health education important? What urgency do we have today?

Today we face a new epidemiological scenario; people and societies have changed their behavior patterns and lifestyle. Previously, the diseases that caused the most deaths in the world were infectious and contagious (malaria, typhoid, cholera, etc.); however, epidemiological studies reveal that this situation has taken a noticeable turn in almost every nation in the world.

Since the 1990s, an "epidemiological transition" has occurred in the countries of the South American Cone, due to new lifestyles that have raised the number of chronic non-communicable diseases (NCDs) whose characteristics are as follows: 1) Prolonged incubation period; 2) chronic evolution; 3) multi-factorial etiology, and 4) the possibilities to cure these diseases are limited, expensive and ineffective.

The most common chronic non-communicable diseases are: Cardiovascular, cancer, high blood pressure, stroke, diabetes, obesity, depression, liver cirrhosis, lumbago, among others. All of them present in a predominantly urban population.

To prevent and/or control these chronic diseases and consequently death, the focus is directed to HEALTH EDUCATION whose action is based on four pillars:

1) Health sciences - What are the behaviors that improve health?

2) Behavioral sciences - How do behavioral changes occur?

3) Educational sciences - How can learning be facilitated?, and

4) Communicational sciences - How do people communicate?

Health Education imparts knowledge whose objective is for people to take care of themselves, their family or community, changing behaviors and acquiring new habits to preserve their state of health. Remember, the biggest capital you have to succeed in life is your health. God says in his Word: "Beloved, I pray that you may prosper in all things and be in health, just as your soul prospers." (3 John 2, NKJV).

It is my desire that, throughout this program, you can learn and reflect on the great principles of health proposed from a Christian and scientific perspective; but the best thing is that you make decisions to change and/or improve your lifestyle, which will help you achieve your greatest dreams[1].

---

[1] Richard, D. Manual de Educación para la Salud, p 2

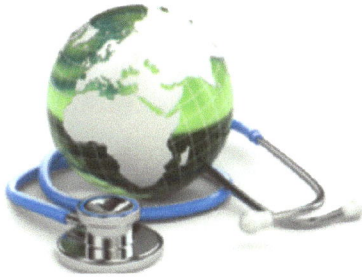

Week 1:
Health condition
in the world

"Happiness, for me, consists of enjoying good health,
sleeping without fear, and waking up without anguish.[2]
" (F. Sagan)

Revealing Statistics

❖ The main causes of mortality in the world are ischemic heart disease and stroke, which caused 15.2 million deaths in 2016 and have been the main causes of mortality during the last 15 years.

❖ Chronic obstructive pulmonary disease caused three million deaths in 2016, while lung cancer, along with trachea and bronchial cancer, killed 1.7 million people.

❖ The death toll from diabetes, which was less than one million in 2000, reached 1.6 million in 2016. Deaths attributable to dementia more than doubled between 2000 and 2016, which caused this disease to become the fifth cause of death in the world in 2016. (Source: WHO)

In the United States

❖ According to the Center for Disease Control and Prevention, the main cause of death in the United States is related to heart problems: according to 2016 statistics, 635,260 people die from it each year in the US.

❖ Then it is followed by cancer, with 598,038 deaths each year, according to 2016 data.

Chronic diseases in the world

❖ According to the World Health Organization, chronic diseases are diseases of long duration and usually slow progression. Heart disease, heart attacks, cancer, respiratory diseases and diabetes are the main causes of mortality in the world, being responsible for 63% of deaths.

---

[2] https://exploringyourmind.com/10-curiosities-about-dreams-that-you-will-love/

❖ However, they are easily preventable, modifying some behaviors in those affected or serving as prevention in those who have not yet been diagnosed, and yet they have become a public health problem both globally, including in our country.

❖ Chronic non-communicable diseases associated with lifestyle and poor nutrition such as obesity, type 2 diabetes, cardiovascular diseases, and disorders in fat metabolism (dyslipidemias, hypercholesterolemia) are now being considered endemic throughout the world.

❖ Considering the high increase of these diseases, in all parts of the world and in all socioeconomic strata, it is important to take measures to prevent and promote health, especially in those people who are exposed to risk factors: sedentary lifestyle, alcoholism, smoking, high intake of salt and junk food, among others.

EPIDEMIOLOGICAL TREE

When we talk about the behavioral epidemiology of the disease, we must remember that there is an individual responsibility in the health-disease dynamic. Therefore it is crucial that, in the face of the rise of chronic diseases, we elaborate our epidemiological tree. In doing so we will discover, in a practical way, what the cause of the death was for our ancestors, at what age they died and if they had one or more diseases. It will also allow us to know if our parents, brothers, uncles, maternal and paternal grandparents and others who are alive are currently suffering from some disease.

Importance

By developing your epidemiological tree, you will become aware of the possible diseases that you might have. So if, for example, in your family your grandparents or parents died of cancer, then the probability that you will die of the same is higher. What can we do? We can improve our lifestyle by changing from negative to positive habits; then the possibility that we will have cancer would be significantly reduced, or at least delay its appearance or in the best case it will not manifest itself at all. Remember, your lifestyle will determine your health now and in the future.

Action for your health

Create your family epidemiological tree. Take two blank sheets, in one place the names of your maternal relatives and in the other sheet the names of your paternal relatives. If they died, put the age and disease for each of them, and if they are alive, put their name, age and what disease they suffer from today. Then evaluate and reflect on what changes you should make in your lifestyle.

——————————————————

Notes

_____

_____

_____

_____

_____

_____

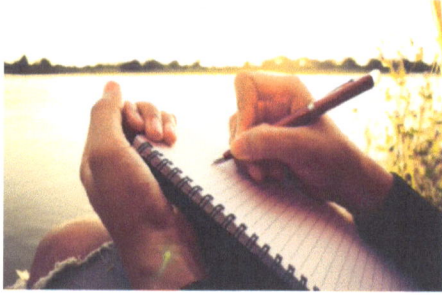

WEEK 2: EVALUATING YOUR LIFESTYLE

*"It is not because things are difficult that we do not dare,
it is because we do not dare that they are difficult.*[3]
" (L. A. Seneca)

Lifestyle

➤ First of all, it should be mentioned that both at the personal and at the collective level, there are forms of behavior that may be favorable to health, as well as others that may be unfavorable.

➤ This derives from the concept of "lifestyle" defined as the "set of patterns and behaviors of a person's everyday behavior."

➤ In other words, as defined by Gutierrez, it "is the way of life adopted by a person or group, the way to occupy their free time, consumption, eating habits, hygienic habits …"

➤ The WHO defines it as a way of life that is based on identifiable behavior patterns, determined by the interaction between individual personal characteristics, social interactions and socio-economic and environmental living conditions.

Benefits of a Healthy Lifestyle

There are many benefits of incorporating healthy lifestyle habits, and these will be fully reflected in the 4 aspects of the human being: physical, mental, social and spiritual.

❖ Prevents problems with obesity, helping us lose weight or maintain the ideal weight.
❖ Increases energy levels to perform our daily activities.
❖ Improves respiratory action.
❖ Helps to have a healthier development and growth.

---

[3] https://www.brainyquote.com/quotes/lucius_annaeus_seneca_107581

- ❖ Increases overall performance: strength, speed, endurance.
- ❖ There is a great improvement in coordination.

Eliminates or reduces anxiety and stress in your life.

- ❖ Contributes to regulate sleep.
- ❖ Improves self-esteem.
- ❖ Helps us face difficulties with hope.
- ❖ Improves our physical image.

Evaluating your lifestyle

How can I tell if I have a proper lifestyle? This is a question that the vast majority of people ask themselves. There are different ways to know, which we will mention below.

Respond honestly to the lifestyle questionnaire. The questionnaires or surveys on lifestyle show us the type of behaviors we have in our daily lives which may be contributing to our overall health.

Visit the doctor and get a check-up every year. Visiting the doctor or conducting an annual check-up should be a constant practice. Many people only go to the doctor when they have extreme health complications and at this stage the type of help that can be given is more limited and difficult.

A complete blood count is revealing about your overall health. A complete blood count is a blood test used to assess general health status and detect a wide variety of diseases, including anemia, infections and leukemia. This laboratory test will reveal if we have cholesterol, triglycerides, sugar, uric acid, etc. in an adequate range and if the different organs are working well.

Stress and mood. If you are constantly worried or stressed, it is a sign that something is wrong, therefore reflect and evaluate what the factors are that are causing you stress and that are affecting your mood in a certain way. Hans Selye, the inventor of the term *stress*, has already said: "a stressed attitude to life breaks us sooner or later.

Mouth problems: They can also reveal how our health is:

- ➤ Cavities: reveal bad eating habits, especially excess consumption of refined carbohydrates and mineral deficits.

➤ Halitosis: bad breath is often due to a lack of oral hygiene, but in many cases it is typical of people with gastritis or liver conditions.

Action for your health

If you filled in the lifestyle questionnaire, congratulations! So now be a health educator agent. Encourage and support your spouse and the rest of your family to stop for a moment and fill out the lifestyle questionnaire. You should also personally assess your stress level, how you are reacting to circumstances at home, at work or in your relationships with people. You should also go to have a dental check-up, to know how your teeth are.

_____

Assessing my stress level

_____

_____

_____

_____

Assessing my mood

_____

_____

_____

_____

Dialogue as a family and plan the possibility of visiting the dentist. Write because it is important to attend to the signs or manifestations that my mouth reveals.

_____

_____

_____

_____

_____

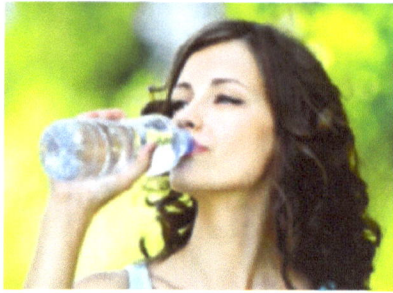

Week 3: Program for Behavioral change

"Habits are like a cable. We weave a strand of it every day and soon it cannot be broken[4]."(Horace Mann)

BEHAVIORAL CHANGE PLAN

❖ Every person who recognizes and understands that it is important to improve their behaviors with regards to health, intends to make changes that should contribute to improving their lifestyle and therefore, their quality of life. However, many times in our eagerness to want to change, we find that many times we do not achieve our goals and we are too frustrated to continue moving forward.

❖ Here is a proposal for behavioral modification of lifestyle. It is based on a combination of planning and programming from health education, theories and strategies for changing behaviors in health, and some principles and techniques in psychology that have proven useful.

❖ Whoever wants to get involved in this change should follow these steps, applying it to their personal experience, therefore, it is important to write out each step.

FIRST STEP

Set your target changed behavior

Select only one health behavior you want to change. Some have the ability to choose two behaviors to change and achieve their goal, but ideally only one. Then the behavior you choose to change will be called negative behavior. For example: I don't drink water, I would like to change and drink water. "Do not drink water" will be the negative behav-

---

[4] https://www.goodreads.com/quotes/7287712-habits-are-like-a-cable-we-weave-a-strand-of

ior and "drink water" the target changed behavior. Now make a poster and place it in a visible place to remind you what you should do each day.

> DRINK 6 - 8 GLASSES OF
> WATER EVERYDAY

SECOND STEP

Make a list of the history behind the negative behavior

The purpose of this analysis is to discover which things from your experience or cultural environment throughout your life have conditioned the practice of this negative behavior. For example: I never saw my parents drink water at home, my grandparents told me that drinking cold water would make me sick, my parents did not exercise.

THIRD STEP

Make a list of the consequences of the negative behavior

Now it is important to answer the following question: What could happen to me if I continue without drinking water? What will happen if I continue without exercising regularly? So if I don't drink water I could: suffer from constipation, my digestion will be slower, I will gain weight, my kidneys will work harder, etc.

FOURTH STEP

Make a list of the benefits of positive behavior

In this step you must find the benefits of the behavior that you will incorporate into your daily life. For example: What benefits will I gain if I drink water every day? If I drink water every day I will: regulate my weight, my digestion will be better, my kidneys will work well, I will control my desire to eat at all times, etc.

FIFTH STEP

Programming of positive behavior

This is a fundamental step in this plan to change your negative behavior into a positive behavior. You need to answer the following questions: How? When? Where? With whom?

How?	I will start to drink 2 glasses of water every day.
When?	At 10:00 AM daily.
Where?	From Monday to Friday in my workplace, Saturday and Sunday in my house.
With whom?	My spouse will call me 5 minutes before to remind me. We will drink water together on Saturdays and Sundays.

After 1 month, after it becomes natural to drink water at 10:00 in the morning, I will now take the next step of drinking 2 glasses of water when I get up, the next month, I will drink 2 more glasses in the middle of the afternoon and so on, until I reach the goal of drinking 8 glasses of water.

Everyone should make a list of new habits they would like to change: Exercise four times a week, sleep 8 hours a day, go to bed early, have a good breakfast every day, etc.

SIXTH STEP

Reinforcing

In the process of changing behavior in health it is important to incorporate some rewards, also known as reinforcers. These rewards are expected to reinforce the new positive behavior until it is established as a habit.

There are both material and social reinforcers. Material reinforcers are objects that you are going to award yourself as a prize. For example: Every 15 days, if we comply with our personal plan, we will eat in a restaurant, or prepare our favorite food.

Social reinforcers are acts or words of recognition that we can give to ourselves, share with others, or receive from others. They can be diplomas, certificates, words of congratulations, recognition, encouragement, or praise. Remember to start with material reinforces, and then include social reinforcers.

SEVENTH STEP

Commitment and Motto

The task is a commitment that each person makes and that inspires him or her to initiate and maintain the behavior until incorporating the new healthy habit. It is also important to write a motto that encourages or motivates you to move forward in achieving your goal.

> I .... aware of the benefits of physical exercise and with the desire to enjoy a more abundant life, I decide today that by the grace of God and the help of my family, I will exercise 4 times a week in this program.
>
> ———————————
> "I CAN DO ALL THINGS THROUGH CHRIST"

EVALUATION

Stop every 15 days or weekly in the middle of your various activities and evaluate how you are doing in your behavioral change program. If you have not completed some days in your plan, try to continue. Remember that changing behavior is a constant struggle, but persevering will achieve your goal.

Action for your health

Developing your behavioral change program is essential to achieve your proposed goals to improve your lifestyle, so keep at it with sincerity and step by step and you will notice how the new habit is forming in your life.

Behavioral health change program

Step 1	Set your target changed behavior. Make your posters and place them in visible places.	
Step 2	Make a list of the history behind the negative behavior	
Step 3	Make a list of the consequences of the negative behavior	
Step 4	Make a list of the benefits of the positive behavior	
Step 5	Schedule the start of your behavioral change plan. Place your plan in a visible location.	

Step 6	Use material and social reinforcers. Write how you will reward your achievements.	
Step 7	Create your commitment on a sheet and write your motivating motto.	
Step 8	Evaluate your program, if it fails, try again. Don't be discouraged	

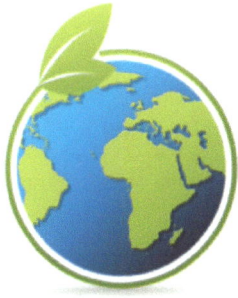

Week 4:
Impact of the environment on health

Everything is with energy

- ❖ According to the US Energy Information Administration (EIA), in 2012, the total primary energy consumption of the world population was 529 quadrillion BTU.
- ❖ 95 quadrillion BTU were consumed only by the United States!
- ❖ More than 85% of current US fuel comes from fossil fuels, a non-renewable energy source that cannot be replaced once it has been used up.
- ❖ The extraction of fossil fuels and other non-renewable energy sources and the by-products left behind cause incredible damage to the environment at an exponential rate.
- ❖ According to WHO, an estimated 24% of the global burden of morbidity and 23% of mortality are attributable to environmental factors.

The environment and our health

As members of this planet, our health is affected by any change in our environment, including flora and fauna.

Trees absorb carbon dioxide that we exhale and produce oxygen for us, but they are being destroyed at an alarming rate. And exposure to sunlight reduces depression, anxiety, lowers blood pressure and helps prevent hypertension.

Air pollution is one of the biggest contributors to many cardiovascular and respiratory health problems and has been linked to:

- ❖ Lung cancer
- ❖ Asthma
- ❖ Allergies
- ❖ Respiratory problems
- ❖ Irreparable damage to plant life (flora) and animal life (fauna)

Outdoor air pollution

➤ Remember that much of the planet's air is inevitably contaminated. Population growth is increasing and we can see in the big cities the tons of garbage they produce. Furthermore, the permanent use of pesticides, dust and ozone, contribute to the problem.

➤ Likewise, carbon monoxide from buses, cars and airplanes as well as heavy metals and chemical products from factories and refineries, all have been adding to pollution and silently affecting our health.

➤ Contamination can harden the arteries: a study by the Southern California University School of Medicine showed that as the levels of contamination increased, so did the thickness of the plaque in the carotid arteries of the study participants.

Indoor air pollution

➤ Sometimes the air inside houses or offices can be as harmful as it is in the outside environment, because the chemicals and bacteria and recirculated through the heating and air conditioning systems of buildings. Chemical compounds, paints, solvents, carpets and cigarette smoke are additional types of pollution.

➤ 30% of all cancer deaths are attributed to tobacco use, causing them to join obesity as the first risk factor related to disease.

Action for your health

Now that you are aware of air pollution and that in some cases perhaps there is little we can do, nevertheless there are actions you can take to reduce or prevent both external and internal pollution.

_____

Apply the 3 Rs in your home, study center or workplace. Reduce, Reuse and Recycle.
Reduce: reduce the consumption of products that are bought and consumed, since they have a direct relationship with waste. Make a list to decrease or avoid your purchase in the future.

_____

_____

_____

_____

Reuse: reuse things, give them as much use as possible before it is time to get rid of them. This way, you decrease the amount of garbage. Create a short list.

_____

_____

_____

_____

Recycle: separate recyclable materials from normal garbage and take it to places where it can be processed.

_____

_____

_____

_____

Remember that it is important to change the air conditioning filter, if you have a permanent filter wash it periodically. If you live near places where smoking is allowed, start a campaign for clean air. No Smoking.

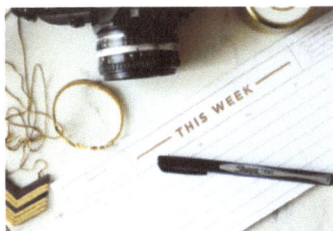

Week 5:
Goals: Assessing Your Health Risks and Establishing Goals

"Everything is impossible – until it's done."
Leonardo DaVinci

The Cold Reality

* 66% of all the New Year's resolutions made in the country are associated with weight loss and improving one's health[5]
* 75% of people stick to the goals for the first week[6]
* Less than half give up on their resolutions six months into the year

Two of the most common reasons why people abandon their New Year's resolutions are: they claim not to have enough time or it's too difficult.

Benefits of losing weight include:

* You feel & look better
* Your overall health improves
* You have greater resistance to illnesses
* You have more energy
* Your mood and attitude improve

Failing to set goals regarding living a healthy lifestyle and making poor nutrition choices can lead to chronic diseases such as: obesity, Type 2 diabetes, heart disease, high blood pressure and other conditions.

What we put into our bodies is what fuels us. And dietary risk factors are the #1 cause of chronic diseases.

---

[5] 1. Journal of Clinical Psychology. (2002, April). Auld Lang Syne: Success Predictors, Change Processes, and Self-Reported Outcomes of New Year's Resolvers and Nonresolvers. - PubMed - NCBI. Retrieved from http://www.ncbi.nlm.nih.gov/pubmed/11920693.

[6] . Sparacino, A. (2016, January 4). The Doctors Office Urgent Care of Paramus NJ - Blog. Retrieved from https://www.onrevenue.us/medexparamusnj/blogcomments?pid=89168.

"When diet is WRONG, medicine is of no use. When diet is CORRECT, medicine is of no need."

Ancient Ayurvedic (Proverb)

The Formula

Set clearly defined goals you can measure and be sure to write them down. Goal setting is a process.

First, create your big picture of what you want to do with your life and identify the large-scale goals that you want to achieve.

Then, break down these goals into smaller targets you must hit to reach your lifetime goals.

Once you have your plan, you start working on it to achieve your goals.

Celebrate and reward yourself as you succeed with the goals you've established.

Goals will drive you to turn your vision into reality.

Action for your health

My long-term goals (3-5 years):

1. _____

2. _____

3. _____

My short term goals (3-6 months):

1. _____

2. _____

3. _____

Steps to reach my goals:

4. _____

5. _____

6. _____

Notes

_____

_____

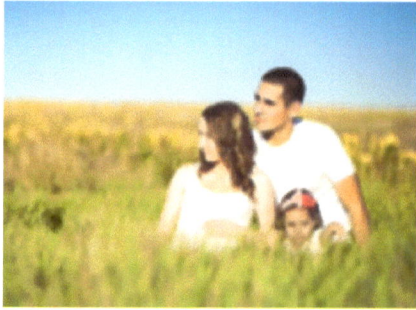

Week 6
Environment:
Spend Time Outdoors

"A merry heart doeth good like a medicine: but a broken spirit drieth the bones."
Proverbs 17:22

We live today with multiple activities and many times we don't have time to spend with our family in outdoor activities. However, there are many benefits that are obtained when performing activities outside the home or office.

Fresh air

❖ We can survive weeks without food, days without water, but only a few minutes without air.

❖ The composition of the air (at sea level) is approximately 78% nitrogen, 20% oxygen, 1% water vapor, 0.97% inert gases - mainly argon, and 0.03% carbon dioxide and others gases

❖ Of these elements, oxygen is essential for every cell in our bodies - for cellular respiration. In fact, 65% of our body mass is made up of oxygen.

❖ The average adult breathes more than 3,000 gallons of air each day. For this reason it is very important that the air we breathe is clean and pure.

Benefits of Pure Air

❖ They improve the appetite and induce a restful sleep - "(The) pure and fresh air … excites the appetite, and makes the digestion more perfect, inducing a healthy and sweet sleep."

❖ Purifies, destroys and deactivates bacteria and viruses, as well as other harmful substances

❖ Increases cellular resistance to viruses and retroviruses that cause cancer and other diseases.

The Greater Light to Rule the Day

According to the Christian Bible, "And God saw everything that He had made, and, behold, it was good." The "good" that is mentioned here is not just the regular "good" as we would normally presume. It goes much deeper than that to cover an all-encompassing and intrinsic meaning of the word. "Good" here in this sense is derived from the Hebrew word towb (tobe). According to Strong's Concordance Hebrew Lexicon, "good" or towb can be described as an adjective in the widest sense, used likewise as a noun, both in the masculine and the feminine, the singular and the plural.[7]

The functionality of the relationships of life here on this planet is so intertwined that without the health of one, another will suffer. For example, sunlight causes the brain to release the hormone serotonin which enhances mood. Exposure to sunlight helps to reduce depression and anxiety and can even lower our blood pressure and help to prevent hypertension. A team of British researchers found out that the nitric oxide which is stored in the upper layers of our skin reacts to sunlight and makes the blood vessels wider to allow the oxide to enter our bloodstream while also infusing us with the beneficial Vitamin D.[8]

Vitamin D helps our bodies fight against illnesses such as tuberculosis, develop healthy bones and prevent osteoporosis and other bone diseases.6 Vitamin D is also a pro-hormone which functions as a gene modulator, thus preventing the formation of cancer producing genes. Adequate amounts of vitamin D is also important for insulin to function effectively and thus reduce the risk of developing diabetes. It is very obvious then that adequate exposure to sunlight is important for health and longevity. Getting 10-15 minutes of exposure to the sun daily will produce your daily recommended dose of vitamin D, which is 1,000-2,000 IU.

Truths About Solar Light

❖ Daily exposure to natural sunlight increases the production of melatonin (the hormone of rest and rejuvenation)
❖ Strengthens the immune system

---

[7] Strong's Concordance. (n.d.). Strong's Hebrew Lexicon Search Results. Retrieved from http://www.eliyah.com/cgi-bin/ strongs.cgi?file=hebrewlexicon&isindex=2896

[8] Reinberg, S. (2016, January). Sunlight Might Be Good for Your Blood Pressure: Study – WebMD. Retrieved from http://www.webmd.com/ hypertension-high-blood-pressure/news/20140120/ sunlight-might-be-good-for-your-blood-pressure-study

- Relieves pain from joints inflamed by arthritis
- Relieves certain symptoms of premenstrual syndrome
- Lowers blood cholesterol levels
- Helps produce vitamin D

Important Facts About Vitamin D

- Vitamin D is a fat-soluble vitamin that promotes calcium absorption and is important in the development of strong bones.
- Other functions in the body include: modulates cell growth (reduces the incidence of cancer), proper neuromuscular and immune functioning, and reduced inflammation
- Several studies have shown its importance in the prevention of heart disease, diabetes, cancer, infections, and autoimmune diseases

We are the Company We Keep

Our environment and those we surround ourselves with impacts our overall physical and mental health. Social influences include: family, personal associations, friends and acquaintances.

People who were exposed to severely depressed subjects over an extended period of time experienced a decline in mood over a six-week period.

Positive social structures can make a very significant difference in our lives.

Helping others has been known to benefit those who suffer from:

- Heart disease, neurological conditions, depression and anxiety
- Stress-related conditions, even cancer

Action for your health

Now that you are aware of the benefits of spending time outdoors, schedule activities that will allow you to enjoy the benefits of the air, and the sun.

_____

How am I sitting right now? Always take deep breaths when you get up.

_____

_____

_____

_____

Is my breathing shallow or deep? Do the clothes I am wearing restrict my breathing?

_____

_____

_____

_____

Have I already (or will) exercised today? Remember that going for a walk, running or practicing your favorite sport will help you enjoy the fresh air, and absorb vitamin D into your body through the sunshine.

_____

_____

_____

_____

Notes

_____

_____

_____

_____

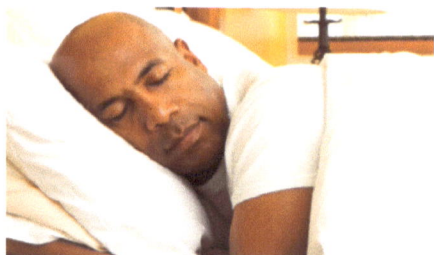

Week 7:
Timely Rest:
Restore, Repair, and
Rejuvenate During Sleep

Sleep Deprivation

Sleep deprivation is a main cause of vehicular accidents in the United States. One study found that driving after being awake for 17 to 18 hours is equivalent to driving with a blood alcohol content of 0.05%. Scientists believe that while we sleep, memories and skills are shifted to more efficient and permanent brain regions. A lack of sleep affects our memory.

The other negative effects of sleep deprivation include: poor memory, loss of alertness, and increased risk of obesity, hypertension, cardiovascular disease, high blood pressure, stroke and diabetes.

Working in the U.S.A.

The United States is the only developed country in the world without legally required paid vacation or holidays. U.S. employees work approximately 20% more hours per worker than employees in Germany or France.

Adrenal Fatigue

Adrenal fatigue is a decrease in the adrenal gland's ability to carry out its normal functions. It is commonly caused by chronic stress from any source including: environmental, emotional, physical and mental stress.

Daily Sleep Recommendations

Teenagers (14-17): 8-10 hours
Younger adults (18-25): 7-9 hours
Adults (26-64): 7-9 hours
Older adults (65+): 7-8 hours

Tips for Getting a Better Night's Sleep

There are a few things that we can do to ensure that we are getting the proper sleep and rest levels that our bodies need to function properly and have enough energy to help us success- fully complete each new day.

❖ We should try to adhere to a timely sleep schedule.
Consistency has been proven to reinforce the body's sleep-wake cycle and help promote a better quality of sleep at night. Try to be in bed by 10:00 pm. The hours prior to midnight allow for more production of the growth hormones. This, therefore, increases the processes of healing and reparation.

❖ Have a bedtime ritual.
Do something that will relax you before going to bed so that you can easily drift off. Forcing yourself to sleep tends to have the opposite effect as it can add stress. Also, warm colored light such as those with a yellowish glow has been known to influence feelings of rest and relaxation in the brain, helping it to unwind.

❖ Daytime naps can interfere with proper nighttime rest. If naps are absolutely necessary or you find your- self utterly exhausted, you should limit your naps to last only between ten and thirty minutes.

❖ Physical activity such as walking, jogging or even simple house-cleaning can help you sleep better at night. In addition to the other numerous health benefits, physical activity can help you fall into a deeper sleep by expending any unused energy that accumulates throughout the day. One thing to remember though is not to exercise too close to bedtime. Try to exercise in the morning or afternoon, because exercising right before going to bed may keep you too energized to fall asleep.

❖ Many people consider stress as the number one reason for not having a quality sleep. There are several ways that you can help to manage stress. Physical activity helps to alleviate stress and the over-production of cortisol during the day which will contribute to better sleep at night. Another good practice is to keep work from interfering with your personal life. Keeping work and home-life separate can greatly increase your chances of falling soundly asleep. Remember, tomorrow is another day. Do not worry about things that you cannot change and always move forward.

❖ Prayer, meditation, and giving thanks for all the day's blessings will allow for a good night's sleep.

In Summary

Please remember that in order for you to attain health and longevity there are two cycles of rest that must be observed: daily and weekly rest. This allows the body to restore and repair damaged cells, tissues and organs. Even God rested at the end of creation week, on the seventh day. He blessed it and made it holy and asked us to do the same. With so much to do and often, not enough time to do it in, we forget about our health as we focus on what all needs to be done. We tend to overthink and overwork ourselves without even noticing the damage we are doing to our bodies and our minds. Although it sometimes proves very difficult, keeping our daily lives organized will help to ensure that we make time for the important things such as our rest, our family, friends, and most importantly, our faith. By following the simple principles and practices of regular rest time like the Bible says we should, we will be able to live longer and healthier lives. We will find more peace and tranquility through the hectic hustle and bustle of each day and we will learn to have serenity in our lives as we were created to. Remember, it is important to take time to rest, repair, rejuvenate, recharge, and refocus. This is a successful strategy for health[9].

Action for your health

Now that you are aware of the benefits of rest, answer these simple questions honestly and find out if you are getting enough sleep.

	Do you sleep enough?		
1	Do I need an alarm to wake up in the morning?	YES	NO
2	Do you feel sleepy while driving short distances or while waiting at traffic lights?	YES	NO
3	Do you run out of energy in the middle of the day?	YES	NO
4	Do you feel irritable and fatigued? (Ask your spouse to respond)	YES	NO
5	Are you a light sleeper and easily wake up with any noise?	YES	NO
6	Are you unable to get persistent worries out of your mind?	YES	NO

If you answered "yes" to any of the questions, you are probably missing sleep. If you are still unsure, try to sit in a comfortable chair in a room in mid-light for 5 minutes. If you cannot do it without falling asleep, it is a sign that you need more sleep[10].

Also, find out what factors are affecting your sleep, stress, pain, caffeine, a snoring spouse, the mattress, the pillow, a noisy environment, etc.

---

[9] Dona Cooper. *Get Healthy For Life*, p. 45,46
[10] Colbert, D. *The seven pillars of health*, p. 51

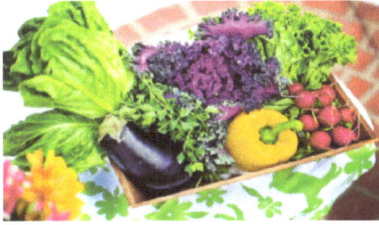

Week 8:
Healthy Diet:
Healing with the Right Foods

Nutrients

Nutrients are substances in foods that provide energy and materials for cell development, growth and repair. There are 6 kinds of nutrients in food:

1. Carbohydrates
   ❖ main source of energy
   ❖ comprised of carbon (C), hydrogen (H), and oxygen (O) atoms
2. Protein
   ❖ the major component in the makeup of bone, muscle and other tissues and fluids
   ❖ essential for tissue growth and cellular repair
3. Fats & Lipids
   ❖ assist in helping our bodies store fat-soluble vitamins and store high levels of energy
   ❖ a healthy diet should consist of no more than 30% fat
4. Vitamins
   ❖ water-soluble (i.e. B1, B2)
   ❖ fat-soluble (i.e. Vitamin A, Vitamin D)
   ❖ 13 essential vitamins are required for the human body to function properly
5. Minerals
   ❖ promote cellular reactions, help to balance the water levels in the body and support structural systems
6. Water

The Plant-Based Diet

Plant-based diets can prevent and even reverse chronic illnesses such as: diabetes, cardiovascular disease, hypertension and more. This diet contains no cholesterol and very few calories or fat. Focus most on nutrient-dense green vegetables with the goal of eating 5 or more servings of vegetables each day.

Leafy green intake is associated with a 14% decreased risk of Type 2 diabetes. Leafy greens include: kale, broccoli, lettuce, spinach, collard greens and romaine lettuce.

Fruits are low in fat, sodium & calories and none of them contain cholesterol.

Essential Nutrients

Essential nutrients provide many health benefits but are unfortunately under consumed in today's society. Potassium helps maintain blood pressure.

Fiber reduces cholesterol, constipation, and the risk of heart disease and diverticulosis. It also promotes proper bowel function.

Vitamin C promotes the growth and repair of all body tissues, helps heal cuts and wounds and keeps teeth and gums healthy.

Nuts & Seeds

Nuts contain fiber, which helps lower cholesterol while anchoring a person's blood sugar. They also contain an array of anti-oxidants and vital minerals such as: manganese, calcium, iron, zinc, chromium and selenium.

Grains

Eat at least 3 or more servings of whole grains per day. Whole grains include: bread, cooked cereal, pasta, quinoa, rice and buckwheat. Grains offer great sources of good carbohydrates which the body uses as energy. However, processed grains are fortified with vitamins and minerals.

Beans, Lentils and other Legumes: The Ideal Carb Source

Bean and legume consumption is associated with reduced risk of diabetes and colon cancer. Beans are a top source of anti-oxidants. If you have trouble digesting beans start by eating small portions to help your digestion become used to them until they cause less discomfort or soak them first to help remove some of the flatulence-causing substances.

Portion Control

Unfortunately, modern packaging does not exemplify correct portion sizes for a healthy diet. A good example of an appropriate portion size is an amount equal to the size of a person's fist for most foods.

Benefits of fruits and vegetables.

Reality

➤ A study conducted in the United States reveals that less than 15 percent of adults in the country eat enough fruits to comply with federal dietary recommendations.

➤ Only 13 percent of Americans consumed enough fruit and only 8.9 percent for vegetables.

➤ Far fewer adults eat the recommended servings of vegetables, according to research by the Centers for Disease Control and Prevention (CDC).[11]

➤ So, in the face of this reality, it is vital that families increase their consumption of fruits and vegetables for many reasons. The advice of the World Health Organization is:

➤ Incorporating fruits and vegetables into the daily diet can reduce the risk of some non-communicable diseases, such as heart disease and certain types of cancer. There is also some evidence that indicates that when consumed as part of a healthy diet low in fat, sugars and salt (or sodium), fruits and vegetables can also help prevent weight gain and reduce the risk of obesity, an independent risk factor for non-communicable diseases.

➤ In addition, fruits and vegetables are a rich source of vitamins and minerals, dietary fiber and a whole bundle of beneficial non-nutrient substances, such as phytosterols, flavonoids and other antioxidants. The varied consumption of fruits and vegetables helps ensure an adequate intake of many of these essential nutrients[12].

Importance of phytochemicals

Phytochemicals are compounds produced by plants ("phyto" means "plant"). They are found in fruits, vegetables, grains, beans and other plants.[13]

---

[11]   https://www.scientificamerican.com/espanol/noticias/reuters/pocos-estadounidens-es-consumen-las-porciones-de-frutas-y-verduras-recomendadas/

[12] https://www.who.int/elena/titles/fruit_vegetables_ncds/es/

[13] https://www.breastcancer.org/es/consejos/nutricion/reducir_riesgo/alimentos/fitoquimica

Science has demonstrated today the importance and contribution fruits and vegetables make to our bodies. There are several foods that can protect against heart disease and prevent cancer, such as:

- Cruciferous vegetables: broccoli, Brussels sprouts, cabbage and cauliflower.
- Umbelliferous vegetables: carrots, celery, coriander, parsley, dill.
- Solanaceae vegetables: tomatoes and peppers.
- Also flax, citrus fruits, onions, garlic, ginger, turmeric.
- Fruits: Apples, grapes, bananas, oranges, tangerines, grapefruit, etc.

Some of these phytochemicals can reduce the risk of cardiovascular diseases, improving blood circulation, inhibiting LDL oxidation, inhibiting platelet aggregation, interfering with cholesterol absorption and modulating cholesterol metabolism.[14]

Avocados

The fats these contain are mostly unsaturated (monounsaturated), and especially note the high oleic acid content. In addition, avocado is one of the richest protein fruits. They are also rich in minerals such as iron, magnesium and potassium

Cherries

Very low caloric intake, high amount of water, contain fiber, vitamin A and minerals such as: potassium, magnesium, and discrete amounts of calcium and iodine.

Banana

Source of vitamins: beta-carotene, vitamins A, B6, ascorbic acid or vitamin C and folic acid. Minerals: high potassium content. It also provides magnesium and phosphorus. High contribution of fiber, with great satiating power. Low in calories (80 Kcal./100 g) and 0% fat. It is the energy fruit par excellence, with lots of important nutrients for our body.

Apples

85% of their composition is water, so they are very refreshing and moisturizing. Source of fiber: contain pectin, soluble fiber. Also contain essential amino acids such as cystine. Recommended in diets and for diabetics because fructose is the main sugar content.

---

[14] Sabate, J. *Nutrición Vegetariana*, p. 340

Oranges

Oranges have a high content of vitamin C or ascorbic acid, fiber, favoring the absorption of iron. Minerals such as potassium, magnesium and phosphorus. Remember, 2 oranges a day provide much of the vitamin C our body needs every 24 hours and half the fiber our body requires daily.

Vegetables

➤ Nutrient-dense green vegetables (green leafy vegetables, cruciferous vegetables and other green vegetables) are the most important foods to focus on for your diet. In fact, vegetables are the number one food you can eat regularly to help improve your health.

➤ Medical professionals generally recommend that a person eat five or more servings of vegetables per day. It has even been shown that these types of foods help prevent and reverse diabetes. A higher consumption of green vegetables is associated with a lower risk of developing type 2 diabetes, and among diabetics, a higher intake of green vegetables is associated with lower HbA1c levels. A recent meta-analysis found that a higher intake of green leaves was associated with a 14% decrease in the risk of type 2 diabetes. One study reported that each daily serving of green leafy vegetables produces a 9% decrease in the risk of developing diabetes.[15]

➤ Non-starchy vegetables such as mushrooms, onions, garlic, eggplant and peppers are essential components of the diet for the prevention (or reversal) of chronic diseases. These foods have almost non-existent effects on blood glucose and are packed with fiber and phytochemicals.

Properties of some vegetables:

Spinach

Spinach is an excellent natural source of vitamins, fibers and minerals, which, compared to meats, provides few calories and does not contain fats. It is also rich in phytonutrients, especially beta-carotene and lutein, making it a vegetable with antioxidant properties that protect us from cell damage. Its stems are richer in fiber than the leaves.[16]

---

[15] Cooper Dona. Get Healthy For Life, p. 58

[16] https://www.zonadiet.com/comida/espinaca.htm

Broccoli

Abundant in vitamins and minerals, broccoli is one of the most nutritious vegetables. A portion of 200 g of broccoli more than covers the daily needs of vitamin C of an adult, since it provides almost four times what is needed. It also fully satisfies the daily requirements of folic acid and two thirds of those of vitamin A. It is excellent for combating iron deficiency anemia and as a preventive against cancer.[17]

Peppers

Contain Vitamins: C, A, B1, B2, B3, B6, minerals: phosphorus and magnesium, potassium, calcium, beta carotenes. Its high iron content means paprika help prevent iron deficiency anemia. Paprika, as a food rich in potassium, helps good circulation, regulating blood pressure so it is a beneficial food for people suffering from hypertension.[18]

Romaine lettuce

Lettuce is the queen of salads, but romaine lettuce is very special because 17% is protein measuring 7.7 grams of protein per head. It is also a complete protein! That means it has all 8 essential amino acids.[19]

Kale

Apparently, this vegetable has a high content of carotenes and flavonoids, powerful antioxidant agents that protect the body from free radicals. Some specifically fight the growth of cancer cells.

Tomatoes

They contain lycopene, a powerful antioxidant that plays a role in cancer prevention. Other powerful antioxidants in tomatoes, such as lutein and zeaxanthin, help improve and protect vision.

Onions

They contain vitamin C, vitamin B6 and manganese. They also contain sulfur compounds, which are said to help protect against cancer.

---

[17] https://www.cuerpomente.com/guia-alimentos/brocoli

[18] https://pimentondemurcia.es/beneficios-y-propiedades-del-pimenton-analgesico-natural/

[19] http://www.todoelcampo.com.uy/beneficios-de-la-lechuga-romana-15?nid=16534

Cauliflower

It contains dietary fiber, which improves the heart and intestinal health. It also prevents digestive problems and reduces obesity.

FATS AND OILS

From a nutritional point of view, fats carry out essential metabolic functions and are important as structural elements and serve as the metabolic fuel with the highest caloric capacity. (1 g of fat provides 9Kcal, compared to 1g of carbohydrates or proteins, 4 Kcal).[20]

However, it is very important to consume the appropriate amount of fats, because if we consume many foods that have saturated fats above the allowed level, our health will be affected in the medium and long term.

➤ The World Health Organization (WHO), the Pan American Health Organization (PAHO), the Danish Nutrition Council and the American Heart Association (AHA) recommend that less than 1% of the total calories consumed come from trans-fat.

➤ It is recommended to keep saturated fat intake to less than 10% and that of trans at <1% of daily caloric intake. The American Heart Association (AHA) recommends reducing the consumption of AGS to 7% (16g / day or 140 calories), AGT up to 1% of total calories and 200mg cholesterol.[21]

Types of oils

Extra virgin olive oil

It is rich in monounsaturated fatty acids that contribute to improve levels of HDL cholesterol (good cholesterol) and triglycerides. Among olive oils, the oil called extra virgin is the most recommended. This is an unrefined oil, with a high content of vitamin E, which fulfills an antioxidant function at the cellular level. It is also rich in phytosterols, compounds that have beneficial effects on the level of blood cholesterol. Its high content of oleic acid makes it very healthy. It is one of the most expensive oils. It can be used as a dressing, in stews or in fried foods, since it withstands high temperatures very well.

---

[20] https://www.vix.com/es/imj/salud/4117/9-beneficios-de-la-col-rizada-para-la-salud
[21] Minsalud. Grasas y aceites comestibles, p 31

Coconut oil

It has antiviral, antibacterial, antimicrobial and antifungal properties. It has been shown that the consumption of coconut oil is good for general immunity, reduces hypertension, helps reduce arterial injury and helps maintain proper cholesterol balance. It is a great source of healthy saturated fats.[22]

Avocado oil

Avocado oil is obtained through cold pressing of avocado meat and is an oil rich in essential fatty acids, omega-3 and omega-9. It is a delicious oil for all those who like this food, and it is very good in dressings and salads.[23]

Grapeseed oil:

It is rich in polyunsaturated fatty acids with a high content of linoleic acid (omega 6 fatty acids). It is soft and easily absorbed. Grape oil is obtained through cold pressing of the seeds themselves and has a high content of oleic and linoleic essential fatty acids, vitamin E and essential fatty acids, also known as Omega 6 and Omega 3. This grape oil is also recommended for people who are following a healthy diet or do not want to gain weight because it contains a type of vitamin E, (tocotrienol), which causes the production of fat cells to be regulated.

Sunflower oil

High oleic sunflower oil is obtained from a specific variety of sunflower seeds that contain a high amount of oleic acids and has nutritional characteristics that make it healthier. It has a higher amount of oleic acids (omega 9) than normal sunflower oil, it is similar to olive oil in terms of its properties, its taste and smell are neutral, it is more stable than other oils so its decomposition is slower, and it is ideal for cooking as it supports up to 200° without being damaged.

Canola oil or raps without erucic:

They also provide linolenic acid (short chain omega 3 fatty acids). Currently, canola with a low level of erucic acid is used, so it does not present problems. In general it is used mixed with other vegetable oils. Its use as a dressing (cold) is preferable. It is not recommended for fried foods.

---

[22] https://aceitedecocos.com/

[23] https://www.enfemenino.com/shopping/mejores-aceites-actuales-s2986078.html

Soy oil:

It has a nutritional quality similar to marigold and corn oil. It is not recommended for fried foods. It does not support high temperatures well, since it is altered with ease, which is why it is recommended to consume it raw.

Peanut oil

It is one of the richest fats in vitamin E and is suitable for all types of cooking because it is very soft and light: sauces, dressings, or desserts, although it is not highly recommended for frying. (better to use olive or coconut). One of the main benefits of this oil is that it does not contain cholesterol, having few saturated fatty acids, and also for its rich, soft taste and a slightly sweet touch.[24]

Finally, evaluate what type of oil you are using. Fats of animal origin have very significant amounts of saturated fatty acids, for this reason it is better to avoid their consumption. Remember that oils or fats of vegetable origin are rich in unsaturated fatty acids, mainly linoleic acid, in seed oils such as: soy, sunflower, corn and peanut. In olive oil there is a clear predominance of oleic acid.

Food or nutrient table and its function

Disease	Food or Nutrient	Function
Anemia	legumes	Rich source of Iron, folate and protein which are used for blood production
	Fruit	Fruits, especially acidic fruits help facilitate the absorption of iron.
	Leafy green vegetables	Green vegetables are a rich source of iron, magnesium and copper, all which play a role in blood production.
	Alfalfa	It contains about same amount of Iron as beef. It Also contains vitamin C which facilitates absorption of iron.
	Watercress	It contains iron, some vitamins and mineral used in blood production
	Red beet	It contains iron and vitamin C and it helps stimulate blood production in the bone marrow.
	Spinach	Contain iron, but slow to absorb. It also contains various vitamins and trace elements for blood production.
	Avocado	They are rich in iron and also contain vitamin C, making it easily absorbed.

[24] https://www.enfemenino.com/shopping/mejores-aceites-actuales-s2986078.html

	Sunflower seeds	They are rich in iron, vitamins B and E. Recommended to be consumed unsalted.
	Pistachio	Rich in iron and copper. Copper facilitates absorption of iron.
	Grape	Grapes are rich in iron and also contain copper which facilitates absorption of iron
	Passion Fruit	It contains iron and vitamin C
	Apricot	They have anti-anemic effects despite not very rich in iron. They help improve anemia.
	Lemon	Lemon facilitates the absorption of iron found in other fruits, grains and vegetables due to its vitamin C and organic acid content.
	Spirulina	This is a blue-green bacterium which was previously considered an alga until recently, and contains high amounts of iron and vitamin B12, although some scientist state that the vitamin B12 is slightly different than true vitamin B12, hence making it difficult to absorb.
	Molasses	It contains rich source of iron and minerals, hence being an excellent replacement for sugar since it serves as a sweetener.
	Iron	Iron is the most important mineral needed for blood production, but non-heme iron from non-meat sources is not easily absorbed. Vitamin C, copper and certain acids help facilitate its absorption.
	Meat	Meat, particularly liver, is very rich in heme-iron, making it easily and readily absorbed. Although meat is useful in certain cases, it is non-essential for blood production.
	Vitamin B12	Vitamin B 12 deficiency causes megaloblastic (large red blood cells) anemia. Poor maintained strict vegetarians are at risk of vitamin B12 deficiency.
	Folates	They are essential in the production of red blood cells. Folate deficiency reduces the number of cells and increases the size of cells. They can be found in legumes and leafy green vegetables
	B group Vitamins	Vitamins B1, B2 and B6 contribute to blood production.
	Vitamin E	Its deficiency leads to production of fragile red blood cells that are easily destroyed.
	Vitamin C	It increases the measure of absorption of iron by double. It also compensates for reduction.

Disease	Food or Nutrient	Function
Diabetes	Legumes	Well tolerated by diabetic because it has high fiber content which helps regulate glucose in blood.
	Vegetables	All vegetables are well tolerated by diabetics because of their low calorie content, hence good for prevention and treatment of obesity.

	Whole Grains	Whole grains are well tolerated and can be used liberally as they help prevent diabetes.
	Fruit	Fruit is necessary in diabetics because of it antioxidant properties that protect against cardiovascular disease. Caution on quantity and avoid dried fruits.
	Nuts	They are poor in carbohydrates and but high in easily assimilated fatty acids and vitamins B that provide energy.
	Artichoke	Its active ingredient, cynarin, has mild hypoglycemic properties. It also contains inulin, a beneficial carbohydrate in diabetics
	Celery	It helps regulate blood sugar levels, decreases cholesterol and neutralizes acids
	Avocado	It helps in regulates blood sugar, decrease cholesterol and also regulates fat composition in blood.
	Onion	Onion helps reduce blood sugar, they alkalize the blood and protect against arteriosclerosis.
	Mushrooms	Studies have shown that mushrooms produce improvement in the disease course, and also contain proteins and group B vitamins. Reduces the need for insulin.
	Nopal	Some studies in Mexico show a drop in blood sugars in non-insulin dependent individuals after consumption of nopal leaves.
	Potato	They are rich in complex carbohydrate and fiber, which make them release glucose slowly during digestion. Caution on amount.
	Wheat Germ	It contains vitamins B1 and E that have anti-diabetic effects. 4-5 spoons can reduce glucose level and need for insulin
	Antioxidants	Protects cells from harm caused by excess sugar. Provitamin A, Vitamins C and E and flavonoids are natural antioxidants.
	B Group Vitamins	Vitamins B1, b2 and b6 are essential in glucose metabolism and transforming it to energy.
	Magnesium	Diabetics run the risk of lacking this mineral involved in insulin production. Wheat germ, legumes, nuts are rich sources.
	Trace elements	Minerals involved in insulin production are copper, chromium and manganese. Chromium is found in eggs, fresh fruits and vegetables, wheat germ.
	Fructose	Found naturally in fruits. It requires less insulin for metabolism thus easily assimilated, but should be used cautiously

Disease	Food or nutrient	Function
Hypertension	Diuretic foods	In some cases, they are as effective as medications of diuretic actions. They function by reducing urine volume, thus reducing blood pressure. They are rich in potassium, fiber and antioxidants

	Fruit	Eating a lot of fruits protects against hypertension. People suffering from hypertension should consume lots of fruits.
	Leafy green vegetables	They are rich sources of potassium and magnesium which help lower blood pressure. Vegetarian diet lowers blood pressure.
	Depurant broth	Broth made with onion and celery and functions in detoxification of blood waste and help prevent hypertension. A half to one liter of this broth is consumed a day instead of water.
	Legumes	Contain potassium, magnesium and calcium which help control blood pressure. They are low in sodium and high in fiber.
	Celery	It functions as a vasodilator and diuretic, thus helps with hypertension.
	Squash	Rich in potassium and low in sodium.
	Garlic	It has vasodilatation and hypotension properties. Need to consume a certain amount to achieve this effect.
	Guava	A few guavas a day reduces blood pressure
	Pear	They have diuretic properties and are rich in potassium
	Grapefruit	Protects the arteries, has diuretic properties
	Milky Whey	It is a depurant and also nutritious. Used in hypertension and other chronic conditions
	Fiber	More fiber in diet, lower risk of hypertension
	Potassium	Potassium rich diet protects against hypertension.
	Calcium	Dairy products are a good source as well as legumes, broccoli, cabbage and nuts. Low calcium can lead to hypertension.
	Magnesium	Magnesium deficiency can lead to hypertension. Good source is found in legumes, nuts and wheat germ.
	Fish oil	It contains omega-3-fatty acids which can help reduce blood pressure. Its use however, must be cautious as it increases cholesterol in hypertensive people.

Disease	Food or nutrient	Purpose
Obesity	Diuretic foods	Their effect helps with the elimination of fluid and sodium and helps with weight loss.
	Pineapple	Eaten before a meal helps curb appetite. Also has diuretic properties
	Sweet Potato	Good source of complex and easily digestible carbohydrate. It produces satiety, and relieves hunger for several hours.

	Cherry	Does not contain fat or sodium, have diuretic and depurant properties. Should be eaten slowly.
	Cabbage	Provide feeling of satiety due to its high fiber and low calorie content
	Broccoli	It has a low calorie content, and also low in sugars. Provides source of vitamins A and C making suitable for weight loss.
	Seaweed	It functions by retaining water in the stomach due to is mucilage structure, hence stretches the stomach and give the feeling of satiety
	Zucchini	It has diuretic properties and also has a smoothing effect on the digestive tract, making it suitable for weight loss
	Asparagus	It nourishes without weight gain due to its high protein and low calorie content. Also rich in fiber.
	Garcinia	Derived from a Southeast Asian fruit, it acts as an appetite reducer.
	Spirulina	Used as a dietary supplement in weight loss, it is rich in proteins vitamins and iron, but extremely low calories.
	Lettuce	Good source of vitamins and minerals but few calories and also produces feelings of satiety.
	Cucumber	Rich in mineral, low in fat and calories.
	Peach	Contains low calories, helps with elimination of acidic wastes. Good source of vitamins A and C. Provides satiety.
	Grapefruit	Functions as a depurant. Contains vitamins A, B1 and C and other minerals and fiber
	Mushroom	Contain low calories and produces satiety effect.
	Cherimoya	Have a high carbohydrate content and produces satiety feeling.
	Pepper	Contain vitamins A and C but low calories and carbohydrates
	Turnips	They have low fat content, few calories and easily digested.
	Milk Whey	Acts as a depurant, rich in calcium, protein and vitamins.

Disease	Food or Nutrient	Function
Cancer	**Fruits** (oranges, lemons, grapefruit, pineapples, plums, berries, guavas, kiwis, acerolas, mangos, apple,)	They are rich in antioxidant vitamins, fiber and phytochemicals that help prevent development of cancers.
	Vegetables (red beet, carrots, tomatoes, sweet peppers, eggplant, onion, garlic, cabbage, cauliflower, radishes, spinach)	The contain provitamin A, vitamin C, and antioxidant phytochemicals that protect against cancer development and growth.

	Whole grains (rye, wheat germ)	They contain phytates that have anticancer properties. High fiber content promotes intestinal motility. Also helps retain harmful substances in the gut and excreted with feces.
	Olive Oil	Contains antioxidants and monounsaturated fatty acids. Studies have shown to reduce risk of breast cancer.
	Yogurt	Protects against breast cancer due to it active bacteria content and lactic acid.
	Legumes (Soy, tofu)	They contain fiber and anti-carcinogenic phytochemicals that help prevent cancer.

Disease	Food or Nutrient	Function
Coronary Artery Disease/ Arteriosclerosis and Hyperlipidemia	Fruit	Consuming a lot of fruits is the best way to help prevent the development of arteriosclerosis. Fruits have anti-oxidative properties and are low in fat.
	Whole Grains	High consumption of whole grains helps prevent formation of arteriosclerosis as opposed to consuming products of refined flour such as white bread.
	Legumes	Have a high content of proteins and carbohydrates and low in fat. Also provide phyestrogen which protect the arteries.
	Vegetables	They are rich in antioxidants and phytochemicals but low on fat and sodium.
	Nuts	They are rich in unsaturated fatty acids that help reduce cholesterol. They also contain vitamin E which is an antioxidant and helps prevent arteriosclerosis
	Fiber	Found in whole grains, fruits, vegetables, legumes. They reduce the risk of atherosclerosis
	Oils	Vegetable oils contain unsaturated fatty acids that help lower cholesterol. They should be used instead of animal oils such as butter.
	Antioxidants	They prevent arteriosclerosis by preventing oxidation of lipoproteins. They include provitamin A, vitamins C and E, flavonoids.
	Garlic	Functions as an antioxidant, preventing the oxidation of lipoprotein, hence reducing the risk of arteriosclerosis
	Folate	Together with vitamin B6, it reduces homocysteine levels which have been shown to play a role in arteriosclerosis formation. Folates are found in legumes, and green vegetables.

Action for your health

Now that you are aware of the benefits of eating healthy, put into practice the advice and guidance offered by the program. Remember that incorporating new habits is not easy. Use and develop the behavioral health change program of week 3 and the results will be great.

> Purpose to return to God's original plan, incorporate more vegetables, fruits and nuts in your diet. It is also important to choose whole wheat bread and thus reduce the consumption of white bread.

_____

_____

_____

_____

_____

> When you buy your products, read the labels carefully and avoid buying products that contain trans fats, hydrogenated fats or butter. Remember that these are very dangerous for your health.

_____

_____

_____

_____

49

Notes

_____

_____

_____

_____

_____

_____

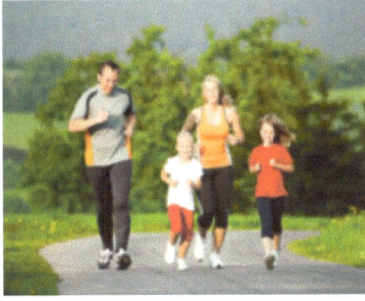

Week 9: Exercise: Regular Physical Exercise is Medicine

Obesity: A National Crisis

Physical activity and exercise can benefit you throughout your entire life! But, obesity has become a National crisis in that 1 in 3 adults and 1 in 6 children are obese. Obesity costs the United States over $150 billion or 10% of the national medical budget each year. Modern trends have discouraged physical activity:

- ❖ Walking, jogging isn't safe in some areas
- ❖ As technology advances, people are finding it difficult to be active with sedentary jobs
- ❖ Children are watching more and more television and playing video games

Small Changes Can Make a Big Difference

A sedentary lifestyle can lead to different illnesses and diseases. Small changes to your daily routine such as walking during your lunch period or taking the stairs instead of the elevator can make a big difference.

Exercise vs. physical activity: exercise is planned out and structured with a goal to improve health or fitness. And physical activity is being active through daily, routine tasks.

Exercise; Not Just Diet

Lack of regular physical activity impairs glycemic control (control of blood sugar levels). Diabetes is only one of the many illnesses that can occur as a result of excess weight gain. One in twelve deaths per year are a consequence of lack of physical activity.

There are typically 3 forms of exercise: strength training, flexibility training and aerobic exercise. Benefits of exercise include:

- ❖ Control your weight
- ❖ Reduce your risk of cardiovascular disease
- ❖ Reduce your risk for Type 2 diabetes and metabolic syndrome

❖ Reduce your risk of some cancers
❖ Strengthen your bones and muscles
❖ Improve your mental health and mood
❖ Improve your ability to do daily activities and prevent falls , if you're an older adult
❖ Increase your chances of living longer

Children and adolescents should get at least 1 hour or more per day of physical activity. Healthy adults should get a minimum of 2.5 hours per week of moderate--intensity physical activity. And healthy older adults should stay active but should follow guidelines as per their abilities and conditions allow.

Frequency: do some kind of physical activity every day.

Intensity: choose an activity that is at least moderate in intensity and also try a bit more vigorous activities during the week. Vigorous activity is the activity that makes you breathe heavily and sweat.

Time (duration): Plan a total time, at least 30 minutes of daily activity. This can be done all at once or join several shorter blocks of 10 to 15 minutes of activity.

Type: The type of activity may include a variety of team sports, individual sports, recreational activities, family activities, active hobbies and walking or cycling for fun and transportation.

Action for your health

Now that you are aware of the benefits and value of physical exercise, decide to continue with this practice if you have already been doing it. If you haven't started yet, then this is the time to start an exercise routine. Remember 4 fundamental aspects when doing so. Frequency, intensity, time and type of exercise. (FITT) Write your weekly or daily challenge.

Frequency

_____

_____

_____

_____

Intensity

_____

_____

_____

_____

Time

_____

Type of exercise

_____

_____

_____

_____

Remember the acrostic FITT, when doing your daily exercise routine and you will be surprised with the results.

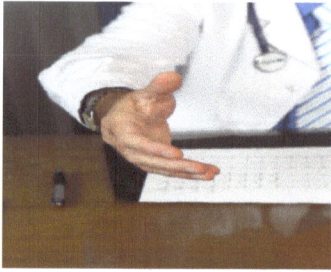

Prevention is ideal

Although disease prevention is ideal, early detection is the next best option. When diseases are detected early, a patient has the ability to respond more favorably to the treatment of choice. Recommended screenings:

- ❖ Initial mammograms at age forty unless a patient displays symptoms that suggest that a mammogram be done earlier .
- ❖ men and women should begin colon and rectal cancer screenings starting at age 50
- ❖ men ages 50 and above should be screened for prostate cancer .
- ❖ both men and women ages 20 or over should be tested at least once every two years for high blood pressure.
- ❖ both men and women should have their blood glucose levels tested by their primary care physician at least once every 3 years at age 45 and above .

Reducing Your Risk Factors

You can reduce your risk factors for cancer and other chronic illnesses and diseases by:

- ❖ Staying away from tobacco .
- ❖ Maintaining a healthy weight for your age, gender and body type .
- ❖ engaging in regular physical activity
- ❖ eating a healthy, plant--based diet
- ❖ protecting your skin
- ❖ knowing yourself, your family history and your risk factors
- ❖ getting regular check--ups, immunizations and cancer screening tests

Know yourself, your family history, and your risks. Get regular checkups, immunizations and cancer screening tests. Find spiritual renewal and reduce your stress levels.

Water: One of Earth's Most Abundant Resources

Seventy- one percent of the Earth is covered in water and it is the most important element of survival. human being can survive a month without food but only a few days without water.

Our bodies are composed of 60% 75% water. It helps us flush out toxins and carries nutrients to our cells. Water also:

- ❖ regulates body temperature
- ❖ moistens tissues in the eyes, mouth, throat and nose
- ❖ lubricates joints
- ❖ protects body organs and tissues and
- ❖ aids in digestion

Dehydration

Thirst is the first symptom of dehydration and if you are thirsty, you are already dehydrated. Increasing levels of activity requires increased water intake. Drinking pure water directly is the best way to hydrate. Approximately 20% of our water intake comes from the foods we eat, and we should get 80% of our intake from direct water consumption. Other drinks may contain high amounts of sugars, preservatives, caffeine and other ingredients harmful to our body. This can cause more dehydration and make our bodies work harder to digest these drinks.

Heat--Related Illnesses

Heat--related illness occur when people are outside in hot temperatures and do not adequately replenish their liquids.

Heat cramps are a result of a lack of fluids and are painful cramps that can occur in the abdominal, leg and arm muscles. If not detected or treated early, a person can end up suffering permanent damage or death from heat stroke.

Heat exhaustion occurs as a loss of water and salt due to heavy sweating. Signs include: headache, nausea, dizziness, weakness, irritability, thirst, heavy sweating, fast & weak pulse and pale, cold & clammy skin.

If someone is experiencing signs of a heat related illness, act quickly and appropriately: call 911 immediately, relocate him/her to a cooler location and loosen clothing to cool their body with wet cloths or fanning. DO NOT give the person fluids at this stage as it could cause medical complications.

Water for Health, Healing & Hygiene

Water has healing properties that have been used for generations to heal a variety of ailments. Hydrotherapy can be used as an internal treatment or an external treatment. External hydrotherapy treatments include: foot baths, steam inhalation for sinuses and congestion and hot and cold compresses.

Water is also used externally to clean cuts and open sores, cool and reduce bruising, ease inflammation and even alleviate insect or animal bites. Aquatic exercises are recommended for senior citizens to increase range of motion without high impact stress on the muscles and joints.

Drink to Your Health!

Eight glasses of water consumption per day is the rule of thumb. Size, activity levels, outside temperature or the amount of heat exposure you get contributes to how much water is recommended.

Foods with over 90% water content include: broccoli, watermelon, lettuce and grapefruit. For flavor, you can add a squeeze of lime or lemon to your water for a low calorie, cost effective thirst--quencher. Filtered water from the tap is also another option.

Action for your health

Now that you are aware of the importance of health exams and the importance of water, do not forget to get a medical exam periodically and make a plan to drink water every day whether you are at home, in your health center work or studies.

Keep a detailed account of your visits to the doctor. Many people have gone for a check-up after a long time without following medical advice and sometimes it has then been too late for their health.

Doctor	Type of exam	Last date	Next appointment

Regarding water: Purpose to continue with your good practices.

Instead of drinking a soda or something sugary, better drink pure water.

Increase your intake of fruits and vegetables, since the vast majority of them have a high percentage of water.

Notes

_____

_____

_____

_____

_____

_____

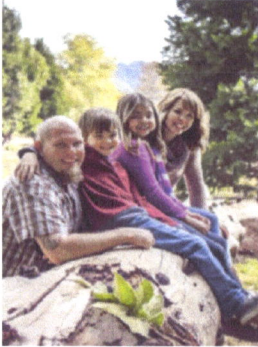

Week 11: Time with Family & Friends

Social Ties: Fundamental to our Health

A huge part of our health is the time we spend with our family, friends and strengthening our faith.   Research has proven a direct connection between the impact that social support has on a person's longevity and their health outcomes; strong social bonds are associated with a 50% increased chance of survival.

Social Connectedness May Predict Quality of Life

Happiness and social connectedness is a stronger predictor of quality of life than the income or educational levels because personal happiness is more closely tied to social bonds than income or education is. In fact, social isolation is a known contributor to chronic illnesses and has been found to be as strong a factor in early death as smoking 15 cigarettes a day. Isolation and loneliness has been known to contribute to poor outcomes in many health areas such as stress, anxiety or depression. Increased health risks open the door for high risk behaviors such as tobacco and alcohol use or a drastic reduction in healthy behaviors like eating well, exercising or getting adequate rest.

What is Happiness?

The ancient Greeks had two school of thought regarding happiness: happiness is a feeling of pleasure and is an emotion AND happiness is about values such as kindness, generosity and honesty and was less of an emotion and more of an idea. However, today modern scientists and theorists in the psychology of this phenomenon are finding that happiness is a mixture of both of these combined. There are 6 domains of human growth important to a person's overall well-being. The first is self-acceptance and the second is the establishment of quality ties to others. Shelly Taylor at the University of California in Los Angeles suggests that stress due to relationship conflicts can lead to increased inflammation in the body, potentially leading to more serious health issues.   Research has linked different forms of generosity to increased health benefits in people with chronic illness, including HIV and multiple sclerosis. When we are generous and give to others, there isa closeness that is experienced by both parties. And feelings of gratitude have been found to be integral to happiness, health and social bonds.

Impact of Social Connections

Social connectedness is more ot a determining factor than previously anticipated for both successes in life and even our mental health. Social connectedness:

- ❖ has been strongly associated with lower levels of blood pressure rates, better immune responses, and lower levels of stress hormones in the body.
- ❖ helps people overcome high--risk behaviors such as: drug and alcohol abuse, smoking and poor eating habits
- ❖ can be linked to improved brain function and a delay in memory loss and social interaction can increase brain activity and keep a person sharp for extended periods of time

God created us to have companionship with Him and our fellow man and without it, we are left with a void. The time we spend with our family and friends will not only prepare us for our journey throughout our lives, but also help us to cope with obstacles and setbacks along the way.

Action for your health

Now that you are aware of good relationships, make plans to visit a family member who has not visited you for a long time. Write on the sheet some people, neighbors or friends who may need your visit.

	Date of visit	Address - Phone
Family		
Neighbour		
Friend		
Someone sick		

Notes:

_____

_____

_____

_____

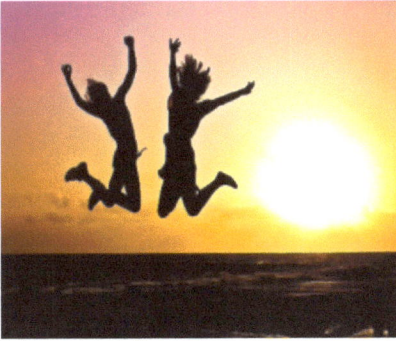

Positive Emotions = Good Health

Certain physical responses such as blood pressure, are considered to be involuntary but we do have a degree of conscious control over them as well. Hippocrates believed that good health was a balance of the mind, body and environment. Many medical conditions that are a result of our mind--body connection are often related to other diseases and symptoms.

Stress is a Killer

STRESS is one of the biggest culprits related to diseases and symptoms. Because of the efforts of a Hungarian-born doctor, Hans Selye, we now have a better understanding of how stress can adversely affect our health. Scientists are investigating whether prolonged stress factors can actually take a toll on the immune system and decrease our ability to fight disease. The human mind can increase or decrease immune function making people susceptible to chronic conditions such as: obesity, migraines, diabetes, heart disease, depression, anxiety, Irritable Bowel Syndrome, gastrointestinal problems, accelerated aging and premature death. A person's thought process could be the difference between health and disease.

Healing vs. Curing

Exercise, prayer and meditation have been proven to reduce a person's stress levels and help them to achieve better health outcomes. Choosing to be happy and hopeful provides whole body "healing" to a person and not just a "cure". Dr. Sandra Levy discovered that hopefulness and positiveness increase survival rates in women.

To retrain our minds and thought processes to think more positively and focus on things such as being happy and hopeful, make time for prayer and meditation. As time passes, we will slowly begin to retrain our mind to a more positive thought process and it will become second nature. It is one thing to cure symptoms, but it is a completely different thing to heal the whole person from the inside out. Having a spiritual connection to the divine can greatly improve a person's outlook on life.

Aging and Living Abundantly

Aging is an inevitable part of life and has long been associated with pain, illness and frailty. However, average everyday people just like you and I are living long and abundant lives even past 100 years old! Technological advances in medicine, healthcare and research have enabled people to overcome illness and disease helping them thrive well into their 70s, 80s, 90s and longer.

Living a long and healthy life is a choice we make everyday. Our habits are the building blocks that we use to build a longlasting legacy. What we put in our bodies is what we will get out of them. Don't put good healthy eating habits off any longer.

Set goals for yourself. Start out with small goals such as buying fruits and vegetables instead of junk food at the grocery store. Try limiting sugary and caffeinated drinks and focus on drinking more pure water. Focus on getting physical activity.

Remember, although making healthy lifestyle choices helps to prevent most illnesses, diseases such as cancer, diabetes and hypertension can happen at any time and to anyone. However, they can be treated and possibly reversed if they are caught at their earliest stages.

Action for your health

Remember that the first step in eliminating stress is what you can control and what is beyond your control.

_____

_____

_____

_____

_____

Gratitude has a very important therapeutic power, when you read the Bible and express gratitude to God, then you take away your focus from yourself and direct it to God that everything can. Then read this psalm and meditate on God's goodness to you and your family.

Read Psalm 103:1- 5

Let my whole being bless the Lord! Let everything inside me bless his holy name! Let my whole being bless the Lord and never forget all his good deeds: how God forgives all your sins, heals all your sickness, saves your life from the pit, crowns you with faithful love and compassion, and satisfies you with plenty of good things so that your youth is made fresh like an eagle's.

Notes:

_____

_____

_____

_____

_____

ABOUT THE AUTHOR

Dona Cooper-Dockery, M.D., is a physician, author, and speaker who has dedicated over 25 years to positively changing healthcare outcomes both nationally and internationally. She is board-certified in internal medicine and holds active memberships in the American Academy of Lifestyle Medicine and the American Medical Association. She wrote the health study series, *My Health and The Creator*, and also writes for and produces the health magazine, *Get Healthy*. Her latest book, *Fourteen Days to Amazing Health*, outlines various success strategies that will empower readers to take control of their health, believe that there is an alternative to medications, change their paradigm, and a live happier, healthier, and more fulfilled life.

Dr. Cooper-Dockery is also the founder and director of Cooper Internal Medicine and the Cooper Wellness and Disease Prevention Center where patients are not only diagnosed and treated using traditional healthcare approaches, but she also emphasizes uprooting the causes of chronic diseases through lifestyle modifications. Her highly effective 12 weeks to wellness program has had significant life-changing results on her patients. Many of whom are enjoying more health with less medication, some have even gotten off medication entirely! These patients have reversed diabetes, improved blood pressure, others have lost weight, reduced cholesterol, or decrease the risk of coronary artery disease and early death.

She is actively engaged in various communities providing healthy lifestyle seminars and free medical care, not only in the USA but also in countries such as Haiti, Jamaica, the Philippines, Senegal, Ghana, and Europe. She is the host of the popular TV show, *Get Healthy with Dr. Cooper*, which airs bi-weekly on two local TV channels. To learn more about Dr. Cooper-Dockery or to get health resources, please visit CooperWellnessCenter. com and DrDonaCooper.com.

www.ingramcontent.com/pod-product-compliance
Lightning Source LLC
Chambersburg PA
CBHW060816270326
41930CB00002B/55